Simple as ABG

by Larry D. Romane, MD

———◆———

INTRODUCTION

ABG stands for <u>A</u>rterial <u>B</u>lood <u>G</u>ases. It is probably *the* single most important test for any critically ill or injured patient. It's painful. It's difficult. And, it's expensive. Yet, even a small community hospital will do a couple thousand every year.

Why? Because <u>no</u> other single test gives as much information about a patient's immediate respiratory and metabolic condition. It's that simple!

Yet, **understanding** ABG's is anything but simple. Traditional textbooks haven't worked because it's like learning to ice skate. If you don't get the first step right, you'll simply fall down on the next one.

Simple as ABG is different! In fact, a field test of students just like you improved their ABG understanding from 55% to over 93% just by reading it! Concepts are simplified and graphs are abridged. Equations may not be balanced and exceptions often aren't even mentioned.

If that much simplification bothers you, your ABG knowledge probably exceeds the scope of this book. <u>But</u>, if ABG's always seemed like a maze of complex formulas, unreadable graphs, and conflicting results, then welcome to **Ted & Larry's** Simple as ABG

About the Editor:

Ted is Ted Heyman, a Florida computer guy. His software helped make ATM's possible for small banks. Now, he's converted Simple as ABG from an e-book format to a print version. He's known Larry since High School.

About the Author:

Larry is Larry Romane, a 4 times board certified, career ER doc from Maryland. He's taught nurses, physicians, respiratory therapists, and medical students. ABG's were always a struggle to teach. Now, step by step, he's made this complex test truly *simple* to understand.

TOPICS

PATIENTS

APPENDICES

TOPICS

Oxygen Transport

(Understanding the BLOOD in blood gases)

If we're going to discuss Arterial <u>Blood</u> Gases, then a few facts about BLOOD seem in order.

Q: Just what makes up BLOOD anyway?

A: Blood has only 3 basic ingredients:

1) RED BLOOD CELLS (RBC's) - you need to understand RBC's to understand oxygen transport.

2) SERUM - this liquid part of the blood contains electrolytes, sugar, proteins, fats, etc. You need to understand serum to understand acid-base.

3) WHITE BLOOD CELLS (WBC'S & Platelets) - forget this, you don't need it to understand blood gases.

When a sample of blood is centrifuged, or just settles by gravity, it looks like this:

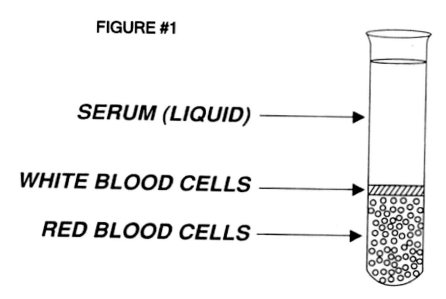

FIGURE #1

SERUM (LIQUID)

WHITE BLOOD CELLS

RED BLOOD CELLS

CAUTION: What follows are not just *some* basic facts. They are *the* basic facts needed to understand blood gases.

Q: Okay, if red blood cells are so important, what exactly is a red blood cell?

A: A red blood cell (RBC) is a tiny human cell found only in the blood stream . It's shaped like a ball that's been flattened on both sides and then dented in. This gives it the most *surface area* for its size and that's essential for its function.

Oh, red blood cells also make blood - you guessed it – RED!

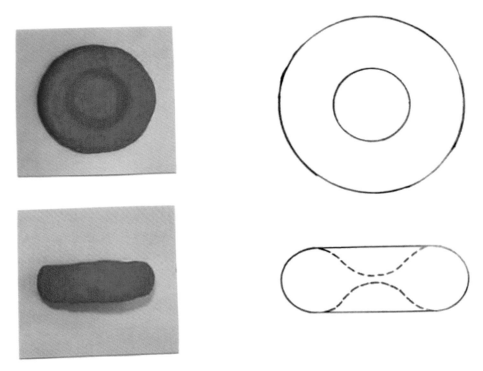

Q: What's the purpose of a RBC (red blood cell)?

A: The ONLY purpose of a red blood cell is to carry oxygen. RBC's pick up oxygen (O_2) in the lungs and transport it to the tissues - kind of like an oxygen delivery truck.

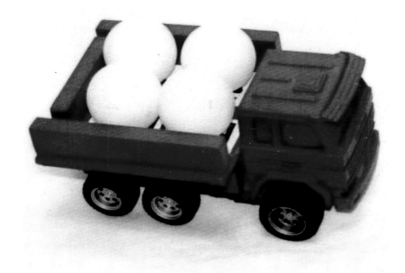

TRIVIA: In fact, red blood cells are so dedicated to oxygen transport, they don't even have a nucleus so they can't even reproduce. Now that's dedication!

Q: So red blood cells transport oxygen, but exactly how do they do that?

A. These pictures are the answer to red blood cell oxygen transport:

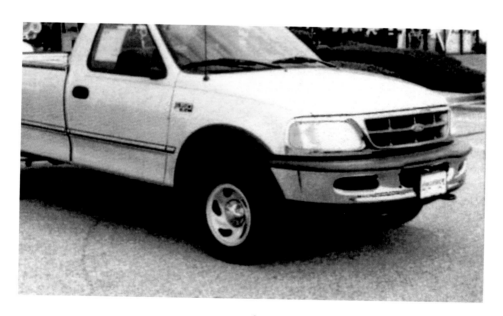

A

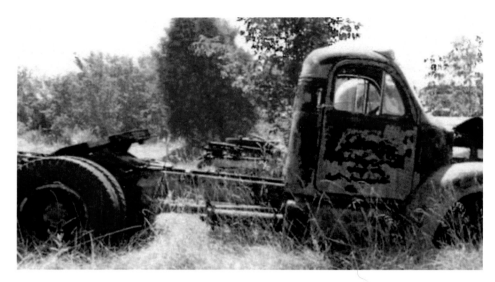

B

Q: What's the main difference between truck A and truck B?

A: Both trucks are made of iron (in the metal compound known as steel). The difference between A and B is RUST!

Q: Then what exactly is RUST?

A: Rust is simply iron combined with oxygen. (Sorry, but we need a formula here)

$$Fe + O = FeO$$

Iron + Oxygen = Iron oxide (RUST)

Q: Iron rusts and trucks rust but do RBC's really RUST carrying oxygen?

A: Yes, but with one key difference. Unlike trucks, red cell rusting is REVERSIBLE. In fact, the iron in the red cell "rusts" (oxidizes) every time it enters the lung. It then "unrusts" (reduces) every time it enters the tissues. This allows pick up and drop off of oxygen.

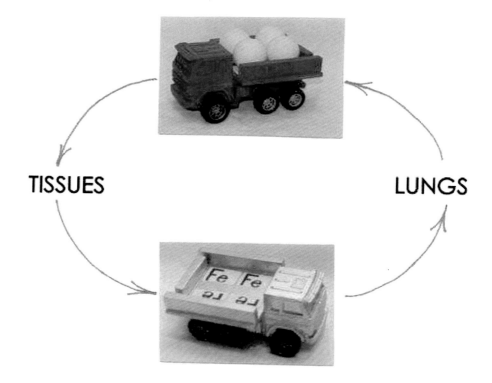

Q: Why is REVERSIBLE rusting so important?

A: Suppose you order a truck to carry heating oil to your home. The truck fills up at the refinery, drives to your home, pulls into your driveway, turns around, and carries the fuel back to the refinery. Result: Unhappy, cold, blue homeowner.

Now suppose red cells drove up to your lungs, rusted to pick up oxygen, went to your toes, DID NOT release their oxygen, then flowed back to the lungs. Result: Unhappy, blue toes.

Q: Is there actually iron metal that rusts inside the red blood cell?

A: No, red cell IRON is not in its metallic form. Instead, the iron is in a complex molecule called HEMOGLOBIN (heem - o - GLO - bin). When these hemoglobin molecules meet oxygen in the lungs, their iron rusts (oxidizes) and turns red.

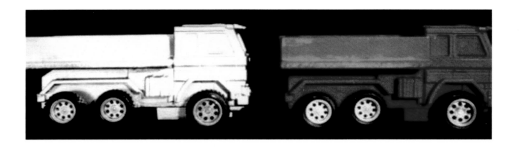

UNRUSTED HEMOGLOBIN   RUSTED HEMOGLOBIN

TRIVIA: Metallic iron is bluish gray. Rust is red. Ever wonder why dead people have bluish gray lips, while healthy, well oxygenated people have red lips? Rusted hemoglobin is the answer. In people, the bluish color is called CYANOSIS and comes from UNrusted hemoglobin (no oxygen).

Q: If hemoglobin is the "truck" that carries oxygen, just how efficient is it?

A: Each iron site can carry ONE oxygen.

There are FOUR iron sites on each hemoglobin molecule. So each hemoglobin molecule can carry FOUR oxygen molecules.

There are 250 MILLION hemoglobin molecules in each red blood cell. Therefore, each red cell can carry ONE BILLION oxygen molecules.

TRIVIA: What is a *billion*? Despite Congressional budgets, a billion is not a small number. If someone gave you $1000 of spending money every DAY, it would take you 3000 YEARS to use up the first billion! The fact that every single RBC can carry one billion oxygen molecules at a time is astounding - and essential to human life.

Q: Does everyone have the same number of red cells?

A: No, different people have different HEMATOCRITS (he - MAT - o - crits).

Q: What's an hematocrit?

A: Hematocrit is a relative measure of red cells. When a blood sample settles into layers (remember <u>Figure #1</u>), the hematocrit is the percent of the sample that is RBC's.

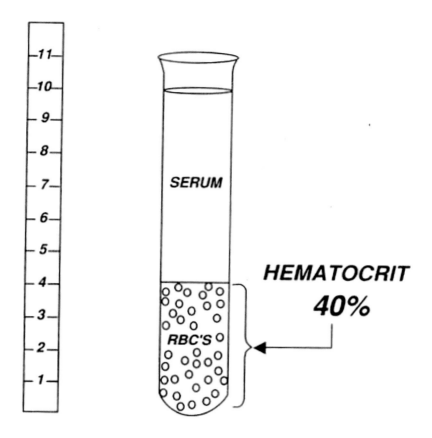

FIGURE #2

Q: What's the NORMAL hematocrit?

A: The normal hematocrit is 40% and often abbreviated as a "crit of 40". This means 40% of the blood sample is RBC's. Any hematocrit between 35% and 45% is normal. Hematocrits below 35% are low which is called anemia.

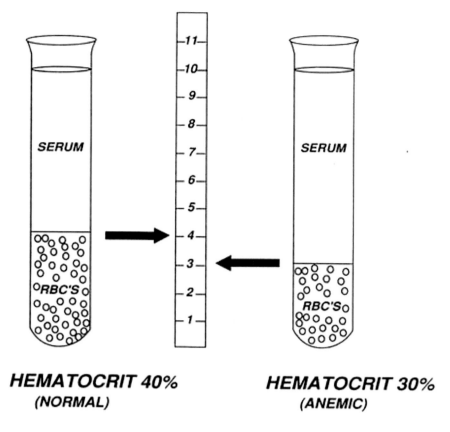

FIGURE #3

HEMATOCRIT 40%
(NORMAL)

HEMATOCRIT 30%
(ANEMIC)

HINT: Remember the MAGIC NUMBERS 35 & 45 (you'll see all this later). They are normal values for hematocrit (35 - 45%), pCO_2 (35 - 45mmHg), and pH (7.35 - 7.45).

Q: Why is a normal hematocrit (35-45%) so important?

A: Remember - people need oxygen and ONLY red cells can carry it. The more red cells, the higher the hematocrit. The higher the hematocrit, the more oxygen the blood stream can carry.

Q: What's the *Hemoglobin* the laboratory measures?

A: The hemoglobin number is another measurement of red cells. It's the WEIGHT of all the hemoglobin molecules in a blood sample. The normal hemoglobin is 12-15 grams (gms) in every 100cc of blood (about 7 tablespoons) . Again, it's a measure of oxygen carrying capacity. Written together, hemoglobin and hematocrit are referred to as the "H & H".

HEMATOCRIT TEST = % RBC'S

HEMOGLOBIN TEST = WEIGHT RBC'S (grams)

TRIVIA: Human beings can, of course, mess up just about anything! Knowing about hematocrits, some long distance runners donated their blood and saved the red cells. Months later their bodies had made new red cells to return their hematacrits to normal. On race day, they retransfused the saved red cells to raise their HEMATOCRITS above normal to carry extra oxygen. Result? The blood was so thick that it sludged. Lucky ones performed poorly, unlucky ones died! The disease polycythemia vera (literally "too many cells") produces the same sludging and the same results.

Pulse Oxymetry

(Pulse ox - the 5th vital sign)

Q: What is pulse OXIMETRY?

A: Pulse oximetry tells approximately what % of hemoglobin is carrying oxygen.

The test is called "pulse ox" for short.

A small electronic clip is first attached to a fingertip, ear lobe, or toe. Each heartbeat sends a pulse of fresh oxygenated blood from the lungs to the skin under the clip. Inside the clip, an infrared sensor measures the hemoglobin that is carrying oxygen as % - the "pulse ox". A pulse ox of 97 means 97% of the hemoglobin is doing its job - carrying oxygen.

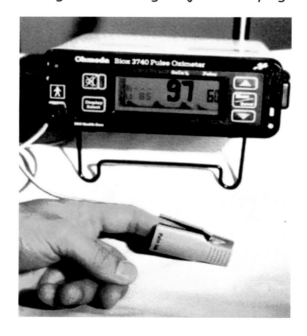

Pulse Ox = 97% (Heart Rate = 60/min)

Q: What are the ADVANTAGES of pulse ox over ABG's (Arterial Blood Gases)?

A: Pulse oximetry has 3 advantages:

1) It's CHEAP. The analyzer and clip can be used over and over on the same patient or on different patients.

2) It's NON-INVASIVE, "Non-invasive" is a politically correct medical term meaning no pain and no needles.

3) It's CONTINUOUS. The sensor checks oxygen on each pulse beat, and continuously updates as the patient improves or deterioriates.

Q: If pulse ox is so good, why do ABG's at all?

A: Yes, pulse ox is CHEAP, PAINLESS, AND CONTINUOUS, but:

1) It's NOT as accurate. Pulse ox readings can have an error of (+) or(-) 5%. The directly measured oxygen saturation of hemoglobin in an ABG is accurate. But a pulse ox of 94% could mean as much as 99%, or as little as 89%, of hemoglobin is actually carrying oxygen.

2) It's NOT actually measuring oxygen. The sensor measures saturated hemoglobin sites, NOT what is saturating those sites. Usually that's oxygen, but some poisons, like carbon monoxide,* can also fool the sensor into a "normal" pulse ox.

3) It's NOT a complete test. Pulse ox gives a good "guesstimate" of oxygen transport but tells nothing about acid, base, or CO_2.

Sometimes, fingertips don't get good circulation. Things like cold weather, poor circulation, and shock can "spoil" the pulse ox. If oxygenated blood can't get to the finger, it can't be recorded by the pulse oximeter.

* Hemoglobin carrying carbon monoxide is called carboxyhemoglobin - COHb. On blood gas reports, COHb tells us what % of hemoglobin is carrying the poison, carbon monoxide, instead of oxygen.

Partial Pressure

(Understanding the "p" in pO2)

Q: What does the "p" in pO_2 and pCO_2 stand for?

A: The "p" stands for the partial pressure of each gas dissolved in the blood stream. It's part of the total pressure of all the gases dissolved in the blood stream.

Q: WHAT total pressure of gases?

A: The TOTAL pressure of all atmospheric gases. That's also known as ATMOSPHERIC PRESSURE.

Q: Huh?

A: The atmosphere is the air blanket that surrounds the earth. It's made up many gases including 78% nitrogen, 21% oxygen, and tiny percentages of other gases like hydrogen, helium, carbon dioxide, etc.

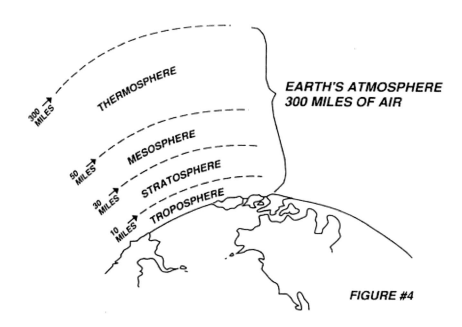

EARTH'S ATMOSPHERE
300 MILES OF AIR

FIGURE #4

Q: Are all the gases equally distributed throughout the atmosphere?

A: The PERCENT of each gas is the same everywhere in the atmosphere. However, near the earth's surface, the atmosphere is densely packed with the gas molecules. At the top of the atmosphere there are very few gas molecules.

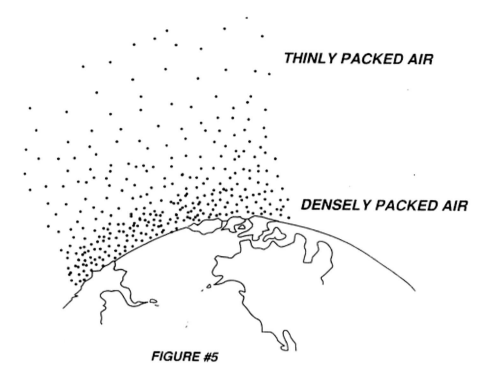

THINLY PACKED AIR

DENSELY PACKED AIR

FIGURE #5

TRIVIA: If air is thin at high altitudes, oxygen is also "thin". Don't try to run your first marathon in Mexico City (elevation 7,575 feet above sea level) or play wide receiver against the Denver Broncos (Denver elevation 5,280 feet - 1 MILE - above sea level). Low oxygen has surprised many a new athlete in these areas.

Let's get back to that column of atmosphere. Whether it's densely packed, or sparsely packed, each and every gas molecule WEIGHS something. That means they all press down upon us. That TOTAL pressure is atmospheric pressure.

Q: How do we measure this total atmospheric pressure?

A: If we're smart, we skip the metric system entirely. Then it's easy. Imagine a square column of atmosphere 1" on each side. Now imagine the height of that column from sea level all the way to the top of the atmosphere. That column is filled with gas molecules and weighs 14.2 lbs.

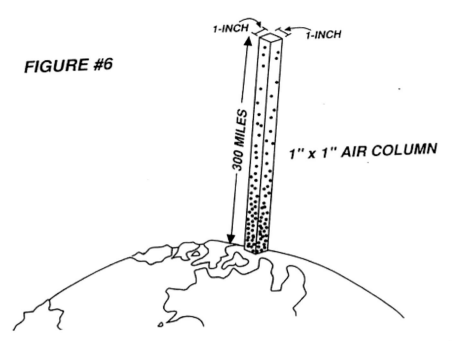

FIGURE #6

1-INCH   1-INCH

300 MILES

1" x 1" AIR COLUMN

TRIVIA: Think we're odd? How come the British list their body weight in *stone*? And sell petrol (gasoline) in *imperial gallons*? That's neither a U.S. gallon nor a liter. Maybe that's why the American Metric Board decided it couldn't convert us. It permanently adjourned itself several years ago.

Q: The inventors of blood gases weren't known for common sense. That's why they used the metric system for atmospheric pressure, didn't they?

A: Correct! First, they concocted the backwards pH scale (see <u>Acids and Bases</u>). Then, they determined that normal atmospheric pressure is 760mmHg, a metric measurement!

Q: What's 760mmHg?

A: mm means millimeter. Hg is the abbreviation for mercury - like in thermometers. 760 means, ah, 760! This time we draw a column of atmosphere 1 centimeter by 1 centimeter (1cm X 1cm) square. Again, the height of the column is from sea level to outer space. This column of gas weighs the same as a 1cm X 1cm square column of mercury 760 millimeters high (about 30 inches).

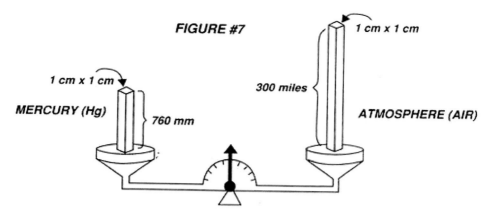

FIGURE #7

1 cm x 1 cm

MERCURY (Hg)

760 mm

300 miles

1 cm x 1 cm

ATMOSPHERE (AIR)

Q: I understand that the atmospheric pressure of all gases weighs the same as 760mm of mercury. What's that have to do with pO_2 and pCO_2?

A: Since "p" stands for *partial* pressure, the pO_2 means what PART of the total atmospheric pressure is oxygen. The pCO_2 tells us what PART is carbon dioxide .

Q: That explains the pO_2 in the air we breathe. What does pO_2 have to do with the pO_2 in the BLOOD?

A: Gases dissolve in liquids. Oxygen is a gas and blood contains liquid (serum). So, oxygen can dissolve in blood. More gas particles pushing down on a liquid means more gas will dissolve in the liquid. So raising the p (partial pressure) of a gas in the AIR we breathe will raise the p of the gas DISSOLVED in the liquid part of the blood.

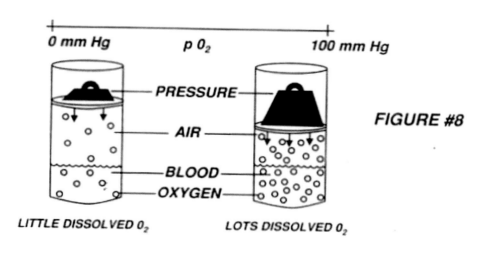

0 mm Hg

$p\,O_2$

100 mm Hg

PRESSURE

AIR

BLOOD

OXYGEN

FIGURE #8

LITTLE DISSOLVED O_2

LOTS DISSOLVED O_2

When we give a patient oxygen, we increase the amount of oxygen in the air he's breathing. That means more oxygen dissolves in the blood, indicated by a higher BLOOD pO2.

Q: If normal atmospheric pressure is 760mmHg, what's the normal pO2 in the blood?

A: The normal pO2 is 80-100mgHg.

Q: Does a pO2 of 100mmHg Indicate a LOT of oxygen dissolved in the blood?

A: No, and this part is tricky. Serum is like a fast moving conveyor belt between the outside air and the hemoglobin. The outside air has LOTS of oxygen (21%). Hemoglobin can carry LOTS of oxygen molecules (1 billion for each red blood cell). But, the "conveyor belt" (the serum) only carries (dissolves) a LITTLE oxygen at any given moment - even when the pO2 is high. That's why we can't live on just serum and need whole blood.

TAKE A BREAK NOW - you've earned it!

The Oxygen-Hemoglobin Dissociation Curve

(The WHAT???)

Q: Didn't you say no graphs and no formulas?

A: How about just one or two graphs and very few formulas?

Q: What is a *graph* or *curve* anyway?

A: A graph PICTURES the relationship between two things. One thing is measured on the vertical line. The other thing is measured on the horizontal line.

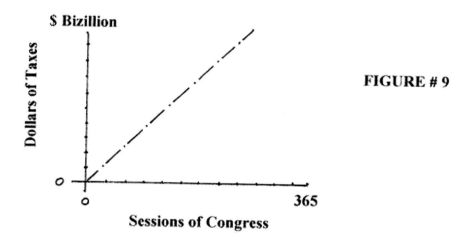

FIGURE # 9

This graph shows the relationship between two things - taxes (vertical line) and sessions of Congress (horizontal line). The line "__.__.__.__" shows that the more times Congress meets, the more taxes there are. Or, the more taxes there are, the more times Congress has to meet - to decide how to spend it all.

Q: What things are measured on the OXYHEMOGLOBIN DISSOCIATION graph?

A: Let's do the vertical line of the graph first. It measures the percent (%) of hemoglobin that is saturated with oxygen. It varies from 0% to 100%.

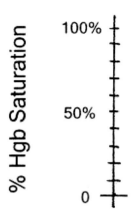

% Hgb Saturation

100%

50%

0

Q: Remember the rusted and unrusted hemoglobin "trucks"? Each truck has four iron (Fe) sites to carry oxygen.

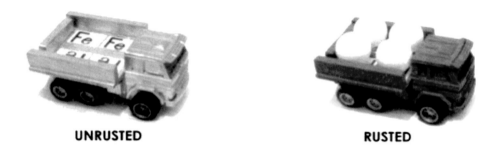

UNRUSTED   RUSTED

REMINDER: You can't saturate more than 100% of the hemoglobin sites because 100% is ALL the sites!

Q: Percent oxygen saturation is the vertical line on the graph. What's the horizontal line?

A: The horizontal line measures the pO_2. It varies from pO_2 of 0mm Hg (NO oxygen dissolved in the blood) to pO_2 of 100mm Hg (normal). Remember the pO_2 is the partial PRESSURE of oxygen. The greater the pressure the more oxygen dissolved.

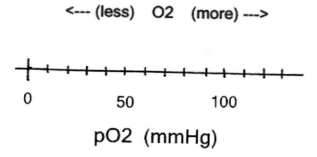

<--- (less) O2 (more) --->

0   50   100

pO2 (mmHg)

Q: Okay, do we finally get to see the famous OXYGEN-HEMOGLOBIN-ASSOCIATION- DISASSOCIATION curve?

A: Sure!

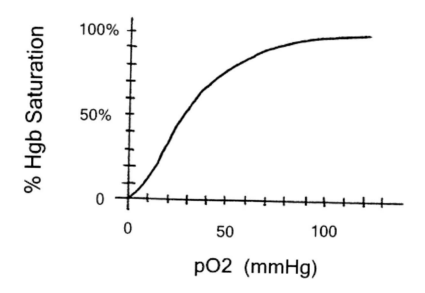

FIGURE # 10

Q: Shouldn't it be a straight line like the Congress and Taxes graph?

A: Nope, that's the safety factor.

Q: What safety factor?

A: Let's look at two points on the curve - A and B.

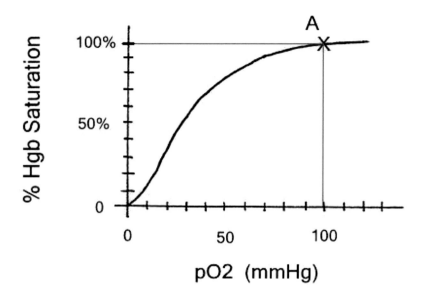

FIGURE # 11

Point A = pO$_2$ 100mm

Point A is easy. If you are healthy, you have a high pO$_2$ - like 100mm. Point A shows that at the pO$_2$ (100) then 100% (all) of your hemoglobin will be saturated (rusted) with oxygen.

Point B = pO$_2$ 80mm

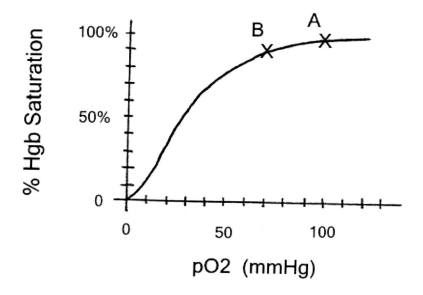

FIGURE # 12

Now, let's say you get a cold or pneumonia. Mucous and germs block up some of your lung tissue. So, less oxygen can be absorbed from the lungs into the blood. Your pO_2 is lower - say 80mmHg (point B) . Because the graph is a CURVED line, you'll still saturate almost all your hemoglobin with oxygen. Actually, your oxygen saturation will still be 98%, even though your pO_2 dropped 20% from 100mmHg to 80mmHg.

Now, suppose the graph was the straight line you wanted. Your illness would drop your pO_2 again to 80mm. Your hemoglobin would now be only 75% saturated at that pO_2. **(Point C)**

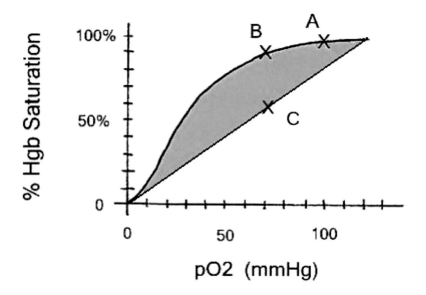

FIGURE # 13

The highlighted area is the safety factor of the curve. It keeps hemoglobin saturated with oxygen even when the available oxygen (pO_2) falls.

Q: Exactly where in the body does this curve take place?

A: Two places:

The TOP RIGHT hand part of the curve takes place in the lungs. In the lung, lots of oxygen comes in with each breath. Atmospheric pressure "pushes" it to dissolve in the blood. This gives a high pO_2. The curve shows that the higher the pO_2, the greater the % of hemoglobin carrying oxygen.

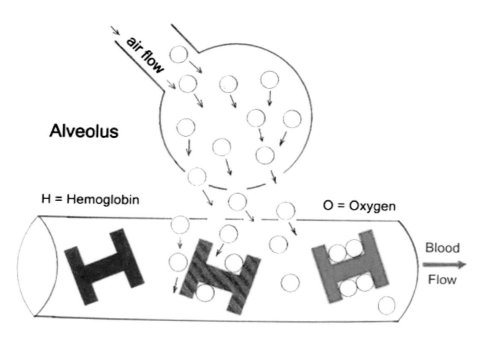

Alveolus

H = Hemoglobin

O = Oxygen

Lung Capillary

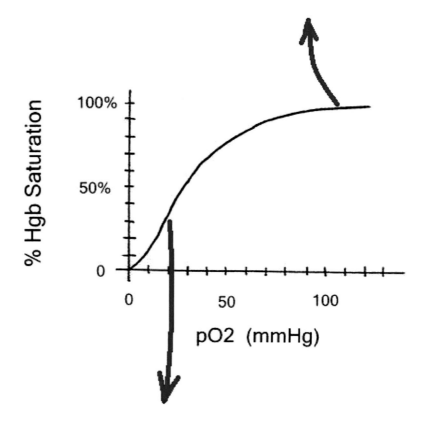

Tissue Cells

H = Hemoglobin   O = Oxygen

Blood
Flow

Tissue Capillary

The BOTTOM LEFT hand part of the curve occurs in the feet (or any other tissue not exposed to air). That means EVERYWHERE except the lungs. In those areas (brain, kidney, skin, etc.) there is very little available oxygen. The pO_2 in those tissues is very LOW. The curve shows that a low pO_2 will cause most hemoglobin to become UNsaturated. It will "UNRUST". Perfect system: hemoglobin rusts in the lung where there is lots of oxygen It then UNRUSTS - unloads the oxygen - at the tissues where there isn't much oxygen.

Q: What clinical value does the curve have?

A: Lots! At any given pO_2 we can predict how much, or how little hemoglobin is carrying oxygen. We can then give patients as much or as little oxygen as they need.

Q: Is that all?

A: NO. Actually, the whole curve can be moved to the right or to the left by various medical problems. That can be a real nightmare. But, it's beyond a basic understanding of ABG's. I've touched on it in the APPENDIX: Shifting The Curve if you are interested.

Q: Want a simple way to memorize the curve? Can you count by 10's?

A: If you can count by 10's, then remember:

A (pO$_2$) of 40, 50, 60 will saturate 70, 80, & 90% of your hemoglobin respectively.

Acids and Bases

(The 'TRICKY' part of ABG's)

Q: What IS an acid?

A: ACID is a hydrogen ion (abbreviated as H^+) or any substance which has a (H^+) to donate. The " $+$ " is important because electrical charges in nature are always looking for their opposite to neutralize themselves - like some married couples we all know.

Q: Well, then what is a BASE?

A: A BASE is a hydroxyl ion (abbreviated as OH^-) or any substance which can DONATE an (OH^-)*. When an acid (H^+) meets a base (OH^-) they neutralize each other's electric charge (+ and -). The resulting combination is NEUTRAL - neither acid nor base.

ACID + BASE = NEUTRAL

$H^+ + OH^- = H_2O$ (Water)

* A BASE can also be described as any chemical that can ACCEPT a hydrogen ion (H^+).

Q: What is pH?

A: pH is the BACKWARDS scale used to measure the amount of acid. It's a 14 point scale that runs from *1* (VERY ACID, with lots of H^+) to *14* (VERY BASIC, with lots of OH^-) . A pH of *7* is neutral, like water.

Q: What's the normal pH of blood?

A: Remember we told you 35 & 45 were "magic" numbers? Well, just like the normal Hematocrit is 35 - 45%, the normal ph is 7.35 - 7.45.

pH Scale

1 2 3 4 5 6 7 8 9 10 11 12 13 14

ACID NEUTRAL BASE

TRIVIA: Why is the pH acidity scale BACKWARDS? Why should something with lots of acid have a pH of *1* and something with no acid have a pH of *14*? There are two possible explanations. First, the inventors of pH may have believed a scale based on negative logarithms actually made sense. After all, a logarithm is the power to which a number must be raised to produce another number, therefore a negative logarithm must be the opposite - whatever that means! The other possibility is that the inventors made the pH scale backward so they would seem to be very clever people indeed - kind of like some computer programmers.

Q: Are there actually ACIDS in our bodies?

A. Yes, there are lots of acids and at least one base in everyone. But, it's easier to remember there are only two KINDS of acid.

Q: What two kinds?

A: There are METABOLIC acids and there are RESPIRATORY acids.

Q: What's a METABOLIC acid?

A: A metabolic acid is any acid that the body manufactures (like stomach acid) or that the body takes in (like certain foods) . Metabolic acids are NOT based on respiration.

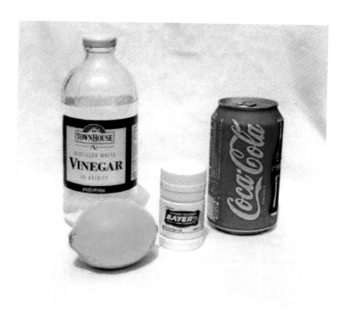

METABOLIC ACIDS

EXPERIMENT NUMBER: 1

EQUIPMENT:
1 lemon
1 glass of water

PROCEDURE

STEP #1 - Taste water, It is neither sour nor tart.

STEP #2 - Squeeze 1 drop of pure lemon juice onto your tongue. Acids taste very sour or tart. The ACIDIC lemon juice thus tastes SOUR.

STEP #3 - Squeeze some lemon juice into water. Taste water again, it's now sour because it has become acidic. The citric acid in the lemon juice just caused metabolic acidosis in the water,

Q: What's a RESPIRATORY ACID?

A: A respiratory acid is CO_2 (carbon dioxide). That's the easy part. Dissolved CO_2 is the only respiratory acid in the body (see Respiration)

Respiration

(Now just take a nice deep breath...!)

Q: What is respiration anyway?

A: Respiration is simply the process of breathing - inhaling and exhaling. Inhaling brings in oxygen so the body engine can burn fuel. Exhaling gets rid of the "exhaust" - carbon dioxide (CO_2) .

Q: You mean "exhaust" like cars and trucks?

A: Sure, CO_2 comes out of your lungs just like CO_2 comes out of your car's exhaust.

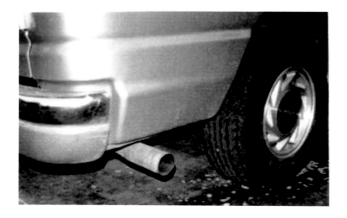

TRIVIA: Most people think car exhaust is carbon monoxide (CO). Actually, it's carbon dioxide (CO_2). A tiny bit of carbon monoxide comes from incomplete burning of gasoline. But, by 1998 emission standards, this became so low that car exhaust suicide is very difficult. Another example is a can of COKE. Open the lid and some fizz (CO_2) is "exhaled" by the can - even at rest. Shake up the bottle, and even more CO_2 is released. When people "shake themselves up" - exercise - they also exhale more CO_2.

Q: I already know about oxygen, pO_2 and pulse ox. Why should I care about CO_2 if it's just "exhaust" anyway?

A: You should care about CO_2 because it's the MAIN ingredient in the acid-base balance of the body.

Q: It is?

A: Definitely. In the body there are two kinds of acids - RESPIRATORY acid and METABOLIC acid. In this topic we'll just deal with the respiratory kind - CO_2. Let's use the COKE example for an experiment.

EXPERIMENT #2

EQUIPMENT
2 small clear glasses
1 can of COKE
1 spoon

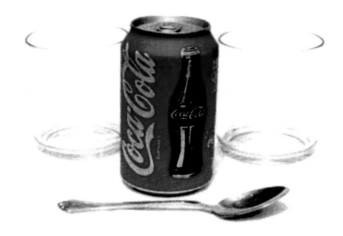

BACKGROUND FACTS

The bubbles in COKE are CO_2.

Acid tastes tangy or sour.

COKE before carbonation is very sweet.

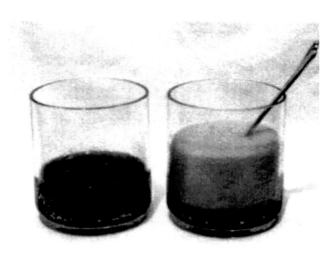

PROCEDURE

1)Fill one glass half full of COKE.

2)Stir the glass of COKE vigorously until ALL the fizz is gone.

3) Half fill the other glass with fresh COKE trying not to lose the fizz when pouring.

4) Taste each glass and decide which is sweet (neutral) and which is tangy (acid).

RESULTS

I'll tell you the answer in case (a) you have no taste buds, or (b) you didn't do the experiment. The flat COKE is sweet and the fizzie COKE is tangy. That's purely because the fresh soda has lots of dissolved CO_2 and that makes it ACID. But, when you stirred it, most of the CO_2 fizzed off into the air. Less CO_2 left in the COKE means less acid and a less tangy taste!

Q: What's the point of this experiment?

A: It's simple. CO_2 dissolved in water makes ACID. When CO_2 bubbles out of water there is LESS acid.

In the body, more dissolved CO_2 means a HIGHER pCO_2 and more acidity. That's a LOWER pH. Your lungs can "bubble out" the high pCO_2 by exhaling. That eliminates acid and raises the pH back to normal.

Q: How much CO_2 do we exhale?

A: Lots. The air we breathe IN has only 0.04% CO_2. But, the air we breathe OUT is 4% CO_2 (100 times as much!).

TRIVIA #1 : Is car exhaust the main source of CO_2 pollution, the Greenhouse Effect, and the dreaded Global Warming? Think again! There are six BILLION people on this planet and everyone is exhaling 4% CO_2, 20 times every minute.

Q: First a topic on pO_2, then a topic on pH, and now one on pCO_2. What's the connection?

A: Actually, there are THREE connections among pO_2, pCO_2, and pH.

CONNECTION # 1

pO_2 & pCO_2 BOTH control breathing. If the pCO_2 is HIGH, sensors in the carotid artery tell the brain to INCREASE breathing to blow off the CO_2. If the pO_2 is LOW, the sensors tell the brain to INCREASE breathing to improve oxygenation. Got it?

HIGH CO_2 triggers more breathing; LOW O_2 also triggers more breathing.

CONNECTION # 2

pO_2 AND pCO_2 are EQUAL partners in respiration. In your whole life you will have exactly the same number of inhales and exhales. Each inhale brings in more oxygen and raises the pO_2. Each exhale "exhausts" more carbon dioxide and lowers the pCO_2. Here's the easy part: it's always 1:1! If you deep breathe room air enough to RAISE the pO_2 by 10mmHg, the pCO_2 FALLS by the same 10mm.

Example:

NORMAL BREATHING - pO_2 = 90 and pCO_2 = 40 (range 35 - 45 mmHg - those "magic" numbers again!).

DEEP BREATHING - pO_2 = 100 (10mm increase) and pCO_2 = 30 (10mm decrease).

CONNECTION # 3

A pCO_2 increase causes a pH decrease. For every 10mm the pCO_2 goes UP, the pH goes DOWN by .08. Remember the Coke? Fizzy Coke has more CO_2 and is more tangy (acid). More CO_2 is more acid, less CO_2 is less acid.

Example:

NORMAL BREATHING:
A pCO_2 of 40mm (normal) gives a pH of 7.40 (normal).

INCREASED BREATHING:
This exhales more CO_2 to a pCO_2 of 30. A pCO_2 of 30mm raises the pH to 7.48. (10mm lower pCO_2 gives .08 higher pH) 7.40 + .08 = 7.48

LESS BREATHING RETAINS CO_2:
An increased pCO_2 of 50mm lowers the pH to 7.32 (10mm higher pCO_2 gives .08 lower pH) 7.40 - .08 = 7.32

Remember: pCO_2 and pH move in OPPOSITE directions. The MORE pCO_2 the LOWER the pH.

HINT: If you think about it, the fact that respiration can influence pH means that a bad respiration could be a pH problem. But, good respiration could fix a pH problem. See Compensation for details.

Metabolism

Q: What is metabolism anyway?

A: Metabolism is the sum of all the chemical reactions that run the body's engine.

Q: Engine? Is this going to be another truck analogy?

A: Sure. A truck engine uses a spark plug to burn (combine) gasoline with oxygen. This produces energy and exhaust.

GASOLINE + OXYGEN + SPARK = ENERGY + EXHAUST

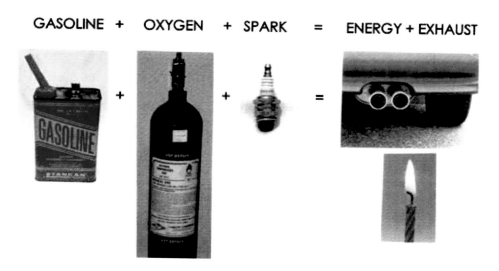

Q: How is that like a human "engine"?

A: A human engine uses insulin (the spark plug) to burn carbohydrates (the gasoline) with oxygen (from respiration). This produces energy and CO_2 (the exhaust).

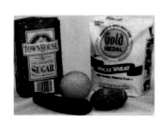 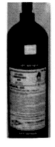 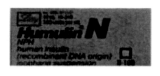

CARBOHYDRATES + OXYGEN + INSULIN

=

ENERGY + EXHAUST

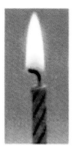 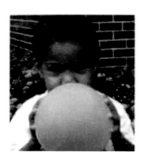

TRIVIA: The human engine burns much cleaner than the truck engine. We ONLY burn the oxygen part of the air - not the nitrogen and other components. So, we don't make nitrous oxide, sulfur dioxide, and the other truck pollutants. Also, we burn fuel COMPLETELY so our exhaust is all carbon dioxide (CO_2) with no carbon monoxide (CO)!

Q: What's the connection between metabolism and blood gases?

A: Some blood gas problems are CAUSED by metabolism. (Just as some problems are caused by respiration as discussed in RESPIRATION.) Blood gases help explain if the pH problem is caused by metabolism or by respiration. Also, ABG's hint at how the body, and the doctor, can fix the problem.

Q: How can metabolism cause acid-base problems?

A: Simple. The body wants a neutral pH. Whenever you have too much or too little acid that's a problem that needs correcting.

Q: But why would you have too much acid?

A: Simple again. Either you ate too much acid or you MADE too much acid.

(1) <u>Ate</u> too much? For lunch you had a Coke (carbonic and phosphoric acids), a vinaigrette salad (acetic acid) and an orange (citric acid).

(2) <u>Made</u> too much? After hard aerobic exercise, muscles give off lactic acid. Diabetics without insulin can't burn sugar. Instead, they burn fat and their "exhaust" is two metabolic acids; acetoacetic acid and B-hydroxybutyric acid.

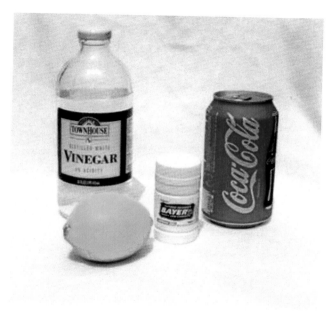

EDIBLE ACIDS

EXPERIMENT #3

EQUIPMENT

2 small clear glasses
lemon or lemon juice
1 teaspoon
1 tablespoon

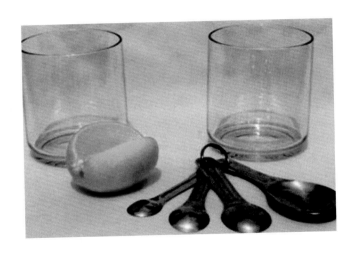

BACKGROUND FACTS

Acids taste sour or tangy.

PROCEDURE

1)Place 2 tablespoons of water in EACH glass.

2)Place 1 teaspoon of lemon juice in ONE glass.

3)Taste each glass. Which one tastes sour or tangy – it's an acid?

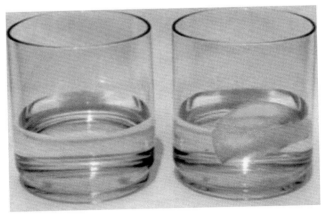

RESULTS

Lemon juice is acid. Added to water it makes the water sour - acid. We did this before. Now stir both glasses like you did in the Coke experiment and taste them again. This time there's NO change in taste so no change in acidity.

Q: What does that mean?

A: You just learned the difference between respiratory acidosis and metabolic acidosis. Respiratory acidosis (like the Coke) is caused by dissolved CO_2. BUT, metabolic acids are liquids, not gases. They need to be neutralized in a different way. Compensation will show you how that's done.

Q: How does all that extra acid affect the pH?

A: Remember, pH is a BACKWARDS measure of acid. The more the acid (H+) the lower the pH. So all that extra acid lowers your pH below the normal pH of 7.35 - 7.45 (average 7.40).

Q: How do we get our pH back to neutral?

A: By reading Compensation.

Compensation

(The lungs and kidneys at work)

Q: What is COMPENSATION anyway? *

A: In biology, compensation simply means returning to balance. In ABG's compensation means returning acid base problems to a NEUTRAL blood pH (7.35-7.45). Compensation NEUTRALIZES the excess acid or excess base.

Q: HOW does this compensation occur?

A: Another experiment is the simplest answer to that question.

*TRIVIA: Remember, biologic compensation is not judicial compensation. The judicial kind is the great American legal feeding frenzy. So, if you eat too much acid at lunch, neutralize your own pH, DON'T sue the chef!

EXPERIMENT #4

EQUIPMENT

3 small clear glasses
Coke
Water
Lemon juice
Vinegar
Baking soda
1 teaspoon
1 tablespoon
1/4 cup measure

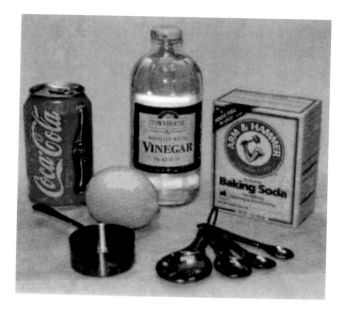

BACKGROUND FACTS

Acids taste sour or tangy. CO_2 dissolves in water to form acid. Baking Soda is sodium (Na) bicarbonate (HCO_3).

PROCEDURE

1) Gently pour 1/4 cup fresh Coke into glass #1 .

Pour 1/4 cup water into each of glasses #2 and #3 .

Add 1 tablespoon lemon juice to glass #2 .

Add 1 tablespoon vinegar to glass #3 .

2) Taste each glass.

Add 1 teaspoon baking soda to each glass and stir gently.

3) Watch results.

4) Taste all 3 glasses again. Still sour or tangy?

RESULTS

When you added baking soda to all 3 glasses they fizzed - CO_2 was released. The bicarbonate of the baking soda attached to the acid, turned it to CO_2, and the CO_2 bubbled off. After the bicarbonate (baking soda) neutralizes them, NONE of the glasses will taste sour.

$$HCO_3^- + H^+ = H_2O + CO_2$$

bicarbonate + acid = water + carbon dioxide (exhaled)

HERE'S WHAT HAPPENED:

Glass #1 (the Coke) had RESPIRATORY acidosis - too much dissolved CO_2. You neutralized (compensated) this acidosis by adding HCO_3 to make the CO_2 bubble off (like exhaling).

Glasses #2 and #3 each had METABOLIC acidosis. Glass #2 had too much citric acid (lemon). Glass #3 had too much acetic acid (vinegar). Again, your bicarbonate (the baking soda) neutralized the acid by forming CO_2. BUT, remember, it ONLY works if the CO_2 is bubbled off - exhaled. So the compensation to correct respiratory OR metabolic acidosis is the same - you MUST exhale more CO_2!

COMPENSATION MEANS FIZZ (CO_2)!

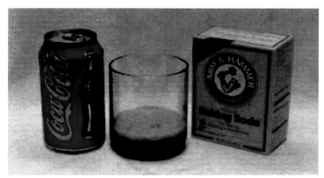

FIZZ FOR RESPIRATORY ACIDOSIS

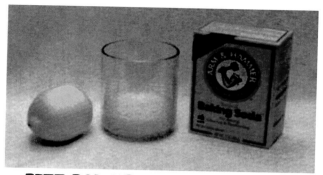

FIZZ FOR METABOLIC ACIDOSIS

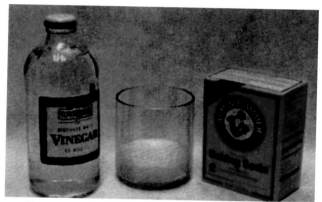

FIZZ FOR METABOLIC ACIDOSIS

Q: I understand the Coke and the vinegar and the lemon but how about BODY compensation?

A: Understanding acid base compensation involves two organs and two rules:

Organ #1 : THE LUNGS - The lungs can blow off (exhale) more CO_2. This reduces acidity just like the fizzing Coke. This is a RAPID compensator that starts immediately. Hold your breath as long as you can. CO_2 builds up in your blood. As soon as you have to breathe again you breathe deeper and faster. That continues until the excess CO_2 that you built up has all been exhaled.

Organ #2 : THE KIDNEYS - The kidneys can RETAIN HCO_3 (bicarbonate) instead of excreting it in the urine. This extra bicarb neutralizes acid just like the baking soda (bicarbonate) neutralized vinegar or lemon juice. This is a SLOW compensation that takes 12 to 24 hours to occur

Q: So the LUNGS are fast compensators and the KIDNEYS are slow compensators. What about the two **RULES** you mentioned?

A: RULE #1

Compensation NEVER overshoots. If your pH is too acidic or too basic it's because of a problem, NOT because you overcompensated.

RULE #2

When the kidneys retain bicarbonate to correct acidosis, the lungs must still exhale the extra CO_2 produced.

(excess acid) + (retained bicarbonate) = (neutral water) + (carbon dioxide)

$$H^+ + HCO_3^- = H_2O + CO_2 \text{ (exhaled)}$$

Q: What kinds of acid base PROBLEMS need compensating?

A: There are four basic problems:

PROBLEM #1 - RESPIRATORY ACIDOSIS - (pH below 7.35). Body not exhaling enough CO_2.

PROBLEM #2 - RESPIRATORY ALKALOSIS - (pH above 7.45). Body exhaling too much CO_2 .

PROBLEM #3 - METABOLIC ACIDOSIS - (pH below 7.35). Body is either taking in too much acid or making too much acid.

PROBLEM #4 - METABOLIC ALKALOSIS - (pH above 7.45). Body has too much bicarbonate. This may be from losing acid, retaining bicarbonate, or both.

The result is still excess bicarbonate.

Q: Should I memorize these problems? What diseases cause them?

A: NO. Don't memorize anything. The following cases will discuss ABG problems in detail.

The APPENDIX: <u>Clinical Causes of Acid-Base Problems</u> lists diseases and causes of each problem as a reference.

Putting It All Together

(Just how DO we put it all together??)

There are probably more *methods* for interpreting ABG's than there are people doing the interpreting. Here's a simple system of questions* that covers all the essentials:

1: Does this patient need OXYGEN?

(Pulse ox < 95? O_2 saturation < 95? pO_2 < 80?)

2: Does this patient need BLOOD?

(Hemoglobin < 9gms? Hematocrit < 27%?)

3: Is there a pH problem?

(pH < 7.35 or > 7.45?)

4: Is there a RESPIRATORY problem? (pCO_2 < 35 or > 45?)

5: Is there a METABOLIC problem? (HCO_3 - < 20 or > 30?)

6: Is there compensation?

(Does each 10 change of pCO_2 give a .08 OPPOSITE pH change?)

7: What's the acid-base diagnosis?

(pH < 7.35) Respiratory ACIDOSIS or Metabolic ACIDOSIS

(pH > 7.45) Respiratory ALKALOSIS or Metabolic ALKALOSIS

8: What's wrong with this patient?

9: What's the treatment?

* For simplicity, you may not need all nine questions for each case study

PATIENTS

(Folks who REALLY care about ABG's!)

Anemia

Tanya "Teeny" Bopper is a 17 year old high school junior. She was brought to the ER one hour after fainting during a one-mile run in gym class. She feels short of breath and the ambulance crew believes she is hyperventilating. She is on day seven of her menstrual period. Her last period was only three weeks ago and this is normal for her. When her mother arrives, she demands that tests be done to find out why Teeny is always tired and out of breath.

Physical exam shows T (temperature) 99.8F, P (pulse) 110/min., R (respirations) 28/min. (normal is 16-20/min.), BP (blood pressure) 110/60. She is of average weight but dieting for an upcoming prom. She is fair-skinned, and possibly pale, but Mom says this is her normal color. To appease Mom, a hemoglobin and hematocrit (H & H), a chest x-ray, and an arterial blood gas (ABG) are ordered.

Results: Hemoglobin - 6gms (normal 12-15gms), hematocrit - 18% (normal 35-45%), chest x-ray normal, pulse ox - 100%. Arterial blood gases follow.

TRIVIA: At T-99.8F, Tanya does not have a fever. The body engine "heats up" throughout the day or with exercise. It is often one degree higher in the early evening (4-7 P.M.) and lower in the early morning (2-4 A.M.). In small children this variation may be 2 degrees or more, which is why sick children always seem to have more fever in the evening!

ABG REPORT

Patient: Tanya Bopper

TEST	RESULT	NORMAL
Hemoglobin:	6 grams	13 female
Hematocrit:	18%	39 female
02 Saturation:	96%	95-100%
p02:	90mmHg	80-100
PH:	7.48	7.35-7.45
pC02	30mmHg	35-45
HC03	29	20-30
COHb	0%	0-1%

COHb is carboxyhemoglobin. It tells us what % of hemoglobin is carrying carbon monoxide instead of oxygen.

CASE # 1 Q & A

To analyze this case, use the questions in Putting It All Together.

Q: Does this patient need blood?

A: You bet she does! With a hemoglobin of 6 grams and a hematocrit of 18%, Tanya has less than half the normal RBC's (trucks) to carry her oxygen. This anemia (low H&H) is probably from frequent heavy menstrual periods. Red blood cells contain iron. When you bleed out RBC's you lose iron. Also, her usual teenage eating habits and her new "prom diet" probably result in poor iron intake as well. It will take months for her body to build new blood, so she needs a transfusion now.

Q: Does this patient need oxygen?

A: Yes! When someone says they're short of breath, give them oxygen. Unlike most medical treatment, it's cheap and easy. Tanya's pO_2 is 90mm which is good but not perfect. Her oxygen saturation is 96% which is again good but not perfect. The other 4% of her red cells (100% minus 96% = 4%) are not carrying oxygen. Since she doesn't have much hemoglobin to rust with oxygen, let's at least be sure she rusts 100% of the hemoglobin she has.

Q: OK, she gets blood and oxygen. What else does Tanya need?

A: First, she needs rest until she is transfused. Next, she needs multivitamins and iron supplements so that she can build new blood cells. Last, she needs to be on estrogen birth control pills to limit the heavy menstrual periods that caused her anemia.

TRIVIA: Currently, the risk of blood born infections (like AIDS) from blood transfusions in the USA is very small. Actually, the risk is one chance in 250,000 transfusions. By comparison, the risk of life threatening allergy from a penicillin shot is one in 40,000 - 6 times as bad!

Narcotic Overdose

James Theodore Junque - "Jimmy the Junkie" to his friends - has been an intravenous drug abuser for ten years. His new "China White" heroin is so pure that he can snort it to get high. Weaker, impure heroin must be injected to get this effect. Tonight, Jimmy decides to celebrate and inject China White into his vein ! Jimmy's dealer - who has advised against this - arrives minutes later. He decides Jimmy doesn't look well. But, not wanting to lose a good customer, he drops Jimmy - literally - at the door of the ER and speeds off.

The nurse finds a stuporous, pale, bluish 27 y.o. male. His vital signs are: temperature (T) 97.8F, pulse (P) 48/min., respirations (R) 8-10/min. and shallow, and blood pressure (BP) 90/60. He has lip and nailbed cyanosis (bluish color), old and new "track" marks from needle sticks, and pinpoint constricted pupils. A pulse ox is 87%. Arterial blood gases show:

ABG REPORT

Patient: James Theodore Junque

TEST	RESULT	NORMAL
Hemoglobin:	11 grams	15 male
Hematocrit:	33%	45 male
02 Saturation:	85%	95-100%
p02:	63mmHg	80-100
PH:	7.24	7.35-7.45
pC02	60mmHg	35-45
HC03	23	20-30
COHb	4.2%	0-1%

Q: Does this patient need blood?

A: Jimmy's life style does not include much nutrition so he's anemic (his H & H of 11 grams and 33% is below the normal H & H of 13 and 40). But, he's not anemic enough for a blood transfusion and that's NOT his real problem.

Q: Does he need oxygen?

A: Definitely! He has 3 oxygen strikes against him:

1. Pulse ox "guesstimate" saturation LOW at 87% (normal 95% or greater)

2. Blood gas O_2 saturation LOW at 85% (normal 95%)

3. pO_2 LOW at 63 mm (normal 80 to 100 mm)

Give him oxygen and you better assist his respirations as well. "8-10 shallow respirations per minute" needs help. "Bag him", don't just make oxygen available by mask.

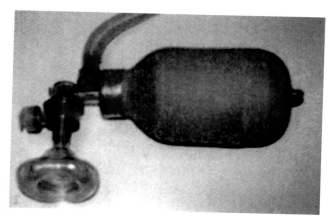

Q: Does Jimmy have a normal pH?

A: No, at 7.24 his pH is much LESS than the normal pH of 7.35 - 7.45. Let's use the average - 7.40 to simplify the math. He must have much MORE acid to have this low pH. Remember, the pH scale is a backwards measure of acidity.

Q: Is there a respiratory problem?

A: Yes, he has RESPIRATORY ACIDOSIS. His pCO_2 is 60mm. This is 20mm above the normal pCO_2 of 40mm. (Normal pCO_2 is 35-45mm. Let's use the normal average (40). Again, it simplifies the math.) Just like the Coca Cola, more dissolved CO_2 is more acidic. Since he's only taking 8-10 shallow breaths per minute, he's not exhaling CO_2 as fast as his body is producing it. Remember that increasing the CO_2 10mm LOWERS the pH .08.

Jimmy's pCO_2 is 20mm above normal. This drops his pH by .16 (2 x .08. = .16). So his pH fell from normal 7.40 to respiratory acidosis of 7.24 (7.40 minus .16 = 7.24!)

Q: Does he have a metabolic problem?

A: No, his HCO_3 (bicarbonate) is normal at 23 (20-30 is okay). But, he will soon have a metabolic problem called DEATH if you don't give him Narcan IV. Narcan is the antidote for narcotic overdoses. That will reverse all of his immediate problems - until next time!

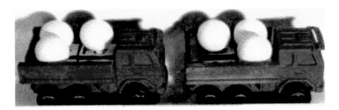

Pulse Ox 75 %

TRIVIA: In this case, any ER doc who needs a blood gas really needs a career change. The method of arrival (dumped), needle marks, vital signs, pinpoint pupils, and stupor make the diagnosis obvious. The blood gases just make it a good teaching case.

Carbon Monoxide Poisoning

Anthony Leonardo is a Chicago undercover narcotics detective. He prefers to work alone for security. His lieutenant believes he works alone to sample illicit substances.

On a cold January stakeout he misses two hourly radio call-ins. Another officer finds him semi-comatose in his car. The motor is running. The heater is working. The paramedics bring him to the ER and suspect substance abuse.

On arrival, Officer Leonardo is stuperous. He is a 42 year old muscular white male who becomes angry and combative when aroused. Vital signs are T: 97.0 (F), P: 110/min., R: 28/min. and snoring, BP: 158/96. His skin is pink, cool, and dry. His lips and nailbeds are bright pink - NOT cyanotic. Lung sounds are normal. Pulse oximetry is 100%.

Even though his lungs are clear, he seems short of breath so ABG's are drawn. EKG, chest x-ray, and urine drug screen are also done. The chest x-ray is normal. The urine shows NO illicit drugs. EKG shows an acute myocardial infarction (new heart attack). His ABG's are:

ABG REPORT

Patient: Anthony Leonardo

TEST	RESULT	NORMAL
Hemoglobin:	15 grams	15 male
Hematocrit:	45%	45 male
02 Saturation:	70%	95-100%
p02:	100mmHg	80-100
PH:	7.48	7.35-7.45
pC02	30mmHg	35-45
HC03	25	20-30
COHb	30%	0-1%

Q: Does this patient need blood?

A: No. His hemoglobin of 15 and hematocrit of 45 are normal.

Q: Does he need oxygen?

A: You bet he needs oxygen! His pO_2 is 100mm so plenty of oxygen is being dissolved in the blood stream. But, his O_2 saturation is only 70%, so the remaining 30% of his hemoglobin isn't carrying oxygen at all. It's carrying CARBON MONOXIDE. ($COHb$ = 30%!)

Q: How come his pulse ox is 100%?

A: Remember, pulse ox is a good GUESS of oxygenation. But, it has a weakness. It reads Hgb as either *free* or *combined* but NOT what it's combined with. Hgb plus oxygen gives a positive reading. BUT Hgb plus carbon monoxide also gives a positive reading, (see Pulse Oximetry).

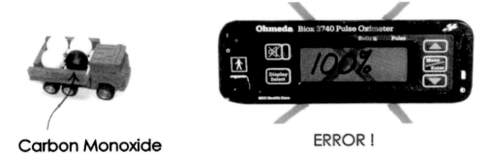

Carbon Monoxide   ERROR !

NOT TRIVIA: Hemoglobin loves carbon monoxide 250 times as much as oxygen. If a room had one part carbon monoxide for every 200 parts oxygen, eventually ALL your Hgb would combine with the carbon monoxide. You'd probably already be dead by the time it reached 40%.

Q: Is the pH normal?

A: No, the pH of 7.48 is slightly higher than the normal range of 7.35 to 7.45.

Q: Is there a respiratory problem?

A: Yes. His pCO_2 is 30mm. That's below the normal pCO_2 of 40mm. How did he lower his pCO_2? At 28 breaths per minute, he's blowing off CO_2 (exhaling) much faster than usual. Why is he breathing fast? Because his body knows he needs oxygen even if the ER doctor hasn't figured that out yet. This fast breathing explains his pH as well. Each 10mm drop in pCO_2 RAISES the pH by .08. He exhaled his pCO_2 to 7.48 (normal 7.40 + .08 = 7.48). (see Connection # 3 of Respiration)

Q: Is there a metabolic problem?

A: Yes. It's called dying! Human beings are aerobic - they run on oxygen. Since carbon monoxide is replacing this human being's oxygen, he's becoming *an*aerobic. This is why his heart muscle is dying (heart attack) and his brain is stuporous and confused.

Q: What treatment does he need?

A: He needs 100% O_2 to try to force the carbon monoxide off his hemoglobin. The increased pressure of a hyperbaric chamber can force HUGE quantities of oxygen into his blood. Hyperbaric treatment is what he needs.

Q: Why not just give him oxygen in the ER?

A: His HMO may not approve a hyperbaric chamber transfer. However, the *half life* of a substance is the time it takes the body to eliminate one half of that substance. The half life of carbon monoxide is four hours when breathing room air. Breathing 100% O_2 lowers that half life to one hour. In a hyperbaric chamber, the half life of carbon monoxide is 23 minutes. That means half the poison can be out of his body in just over 20 minutes. Where would you want to be treated? At home? In the ER? In the hyperbaric chamber? At your HMO's corporate headquarters? Your choice?

TRIVIA: His lips and nailbeds aren't cyanotic (blue) because when hemoglobin combines with CO, it forms a very bright red compound called carboxyhemoglobin which makes them appear *cherry red*.

Aspirin Overdose

Melissa M. is a 42 year old manic-depressive bipolar patient and a frequent ER visitor. She is often nasty, always demanding, and never compliant with psychiatric follow-up. A traffic dispute today led to alcohol tonight, followed by anger, and topped with depression. Paramedics were called when she trashed most of her apartment. **Dozens** of over-the-counter and prescription drugs were found at the scene.

On arrival, Melissa is combative and restrained to the stretcher. She is talking and acting "crazy". Vital signs are T: 97.8F, P: 120/min., R: 32/min. and deep, BP 148/96. Pulse ox is 100% when it can be kept on her finger. She has alcohol on her breath. Crying that she wants "to end it all" then threatening lawsuit if she's not discharged, Melissa is clearly confused. Her physical exam is otherwise negative.

Because of her behavior and abnormal vital signs, tests are ordered. ABG's, urine drug screen, alcohol/Tylenol/aspirin levels are sent off. The alcohol level is 150 (100 is legally drunk). Urine drug screen and Tylenol levels are negative. The aspirin level is 80mg % (10-20 is the normal therapeutic dose). Her blood gases show:

ABG REPORT

Patient: Melissa M.

TEST	RESULT	NORMAL
Hemoglobin:	12 grams	13 female
Hematocrit:	36%	39 female
02 Saturation:	100%	95-100%
p02:	105mmHg	80-100
PH:	7.48	7.35-7.45
pC02:	25mmHg	35-45
HC03	10	20-30
COHb	3%	0-1%

Q: Does this patient need blood?

A: No, a Hgb of 12 and a Hct of 36% is normal. Women usually have a lower H & H than men.

Q: Does she need oxygen?

A: No. Her pulse ox of 100% is confirmed by her blood gases. The O_2 saturation is 100% and the pO_2 is 105mm - both normal. Some of her hemoglobin is NOT carrying oxygen since her COHb shows 3%. This means 3% of her hemoglobin is carrying carbon monoxide. (From her 2 pack a day smoking habit) Cigarette smokers "normally" have 3 to 6% carbon monoxide poisoning.

Q: Is her pH normal?

A: Maybe.

Q: You said a normal pH is 7.35 to 7.45. Her pH is 7.48. Isn't that abnormal?

A: Maybe. Her pH is 7.48 which is SLIGHTLY high. So, either she has a slight acid base problem, or she has a BIG acid base problem pulling her in opposite directions. If you have too much acid for one reason, and too little acid for another reason, you pH may SEEM normal.

Q: What?

A: Just because the pH is almost normal doesn't rule out an acid base problem. Her pCO_2 is 25mm (low), so her pH should be high - 7.52. Remember, a 10 point change of CO_2 gives an OPPOSITE change of .08 in pH. (see Connection # 3 of Respiration) Melissa's pCO_2 dropped 15 points from normal 40 to 25. So, her pH should have gone up by .12 (.08 X 1.5 = .12). Her pH should have been 7.52 instead of the 7.48 that showed on the ABG's. Something is wrong and that something is ASPIRIN POISONING. A level of 80mg % is life threatening.

Q: Why?

A: Aspirin is a strange poison. First, aspirin is acetylsalicilic ACID so when you take too much, it adds acid to the blood. Second, aspirin alters normal aerobic metabolism making more acid in the blood. That means ACIDOSIS with a low pH. BUT, aspirin also directly stimulates the brain to over-breathe. This over-breathing decreased Melissa's pCO_2 to 25mm. Since CO_2 is acid, lowering that CO_2 should have raised her pH to 7.52. But, again, her pH is really 7.48.

Q: Why?

A: Because the metabolic acidosis effects of the aspirin are competing with the respiratory alkalosis effects (over-breathing). This causes a MIXED problem.

Q: Is that mixed as in "mixed up" - like anybody trying to read this?

A: No, that's MIXED as in a mixed acid problem and base problem in the same patient. It's NOT compensation, since the kidneys take 24 hours to compensate and compensation never overshoots. (A pH of 7.48 is not normal)

Q: What is her ABG diagnosis?

A: This patient has a mixed problem: METABOLIC ACIDOSIS and RESPIRATORY ALKALOSIS.

Q: What can be done?

A: First, insure ABC's of resuscitation: Airway, breathing, and circulation. Then, the stomach can be pumped out of the remaining aspirin. Next, oral charcoal will prevent absorption of aspirin still in the intestine. But, 80mg % aspirin is a dangerous OD (overdose). It can cause ulcers, bleeding, confusion, seizures, dehydration (as the kidneys try to excrete it), low blood sugar (as the aspirin alters normal metabolism), and BOTH metabolic acidosis and respiratory alkalosis. So, we need to get rid of the aspirin. The kidneys excrete it best when the blood stream is alkaline (pH over 7.50). So, while giving IV fluids and sugar we'll add bicarbonate to the IV to keep the pH above that number. A dialysis doctor should also be consulted.

Emphysema

William S. Marlborough, III is a 63 year old commodities trader. This multi-millionaire made his fortune in tobacco futures. Born in North Carolina, he has gone through four wives, numerous holding companies, and three packs of unfiltered cigarettes every day since his teens. In the last year, he has also gone through 2 liter/min. of home oxygen for his emphysema. He told his doctor he had stopped smoking.

Today he became SOB (short of breath) enroute to a business meeting. His chauffeur brought him to the ER at noon. His chief complaint is "I have a cold and my doctor gave me the wrong antibiotic." For three days he's had increasing cough, phlegm, and SOB despite upping his home oxygen to 3 liter/min. He feels weak and feverish but "must" be at his meeting by 1:00.

On arrival, he is acutely SOB. His vital signs are T: 102.0 F, P: 120/min. and irregular, R: 20/min. and labored, BP: 168/88. His skin is hot and damp and his lips and nails are bluish (cyanotic). Listening to his chest, you hear scattered wheezes and very decreased breath sounds in both lungs. His pulse ox is only 85% despite his 3 1/min. oxygen.

Regardless of his pressing meeting, a CBC, blood gases, EKG, and chest x-ray are done. The CBC shows a hemoglobin of 16gms and a hematocrit of 48%. EKG shows a fast heart rate with extra beats. Chest x-ray shows emphysema and pneumonia. His ABG's are:

Patient: William S. Marlborough, III

TEST	RESULT	NORMAL
Hemoglobin:	16 grams	15 male
Hematocrit:	48%	45 male
02 Saturation:	78%	95-100%
p02:	54mmHg	80-100
PH:	7.32	7.35-7.45
pC02	60mmHg	35-45
HC03	33	20-30
COHb	4.2%	0-1%

Q: Does this patient need blood?

A: No. In fact, his H & H of 16 grams and 48% is HIGHER than usual. He's been so low on oxygen for so long, his body thought that more hemoglobin might help carry more of the oxygen. But, emphysema, not hemoglobin, is his problem.

Q: Does he need oxygen?

A: WAIT A MINUTE! You've already read two-thirds of this book and you ask if he needs oxygen? He's BLUE: he's short of breath; his pulse ox is 85%; his pO_2 is 40mm. He certainly does need oxygen.

Q: How MUCH oxygen does he need?

A: That's the problem. He's already on three liters of oxygen. That's about 50% more than you or I get breathing room air. But, wait a minute before you change him to pure oxygen at 100%. Remember there are two respiratory drives - high CO_2 and low O_2- (see <u>Connection # 1 of Respiration</u>) Emphysema patients can't EXHALE very well. So, over the years, they retain the CO_2 that should have been exhaled. Their pCO_2 gradually rises and their brain gets used to it. High CO_2 no longer drives them to breathe. Only the "drive" of a LOW oxygen keeps them going. Problem: His low pO_2 proves his vital organs need more oxygen. But if we increase his pO_2 to normal, he'll have NO respiratory drive. He'll gradually drift off to sleep and forget to breathe - and die! Let's raise his oxygen but be ready with a respirator to breathe for him if his breathing slows down.

Q: Is his pH normal?

A: No. His pH is 7.32 which is lower than the normal of 7.40. Since a low pH means ACIDOSIS, he's in acidosis, but it's not as bad as it could be.

Q: Why not?

A: Let's look at his pCO_2 and his HCO_3 and see why it could be worse.

Q: Isn't this a respiratory problem? Why worry about HCO_3 which is metabolic?

A: Of course it's a respiratory problem. He has emphysema AND pneumonia -that's a big respiratory problem.

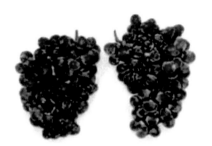
Normal Lungs

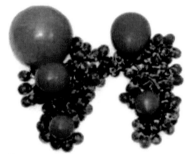
Emphysema Lungs with Blebs

His pCO_2 is 60mm. That's high. CO_2 exchange is a respiratory function.

CO_2 dissolves to make acid. So, he has RESPIRATORY ACIDOSIS.

Q: Well how could it be worse? Does he have a metabolic problem as well?

A: No. He has a metabolic SOLUTION, not a problem. At least it's a partial solution. His pCO_2 (acid) is high but so is his HCO_3 (base) at 33. Over the years of emphysema, his CO_2 kept creeping up as his ability to exhale dwindled. More CO_2 meant more acid in his blood. The kidneys sensed this, and began to retain more HCO_3 instead of excreting it out as usual. That's why his HCO_3 is higher at 33. It's also why his pH is NOT as low (acidic) as you'd expect.

Q: Are you sure?

A: Of course I'm sure, I made up the case. His pCO_2 is elevated to 60mm. That's 20mm above normal pCO_2 of 40. Remember: Each 10mm increase in pCO_2 lowers the pH by .08. So, his pH should be lowered by 2 X .08 = .16 to a pH of 7.24 (7.40 minus .16 = 7.24). But his ABG's show a more normal (higher) pH of 7.32. His high HCO_3 (33) retained by his kidneys, neutralized (COMPENSATED), so he's not as acidotic as he could be.

Q: What is his ABG diagnosis?

A: He's in PARTIALLY COMPENSATED RESPIRATORY ACIDOSIS.

Q: What does he need for treatment?

A: He needs hospitalization, IV antibiotics, increased O_2, and possibly a mechanical respirator with a tube in his trachea (windpipe). We probably can't increase his O_2 enough, without ending his respiratory drive.

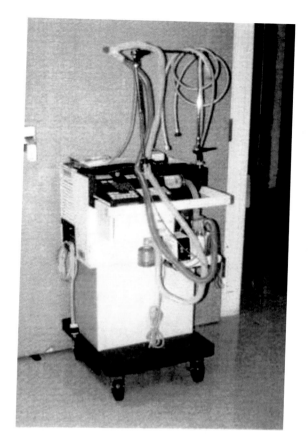

Mechanical Respirator

TRIVIA: Why is his COHb 4.2, even though he stopped smoking? The answer is simply that he never stopped. Despite the claims of the American Tobacco Lobby, cigarettes kill more than 1000 people per day and nicotine is addictive. Simply telling patients like this to stop smoking is rarely successful.

Hyperventilation Syndrome

Annie Hood is a 20 year old college sophomore. She's a vegetarian, a straight A student, and "pretty nervous" according to her friends. Last night, despite weeks of preparation, she drank lots of coffee to stay up all night studying for a test. Shortly after the test began, she started to feel breathless. Fearing she wasn't getting enough air she began to breathe deeper and faster. Within minutes her chest became tight and her mouth dried out. Her arms and legs became numb and tingly and then her hands went into spasm. She felt light-headed and nearly passed out.

Annie arrived in the ER by ambulance. She is acutely short of breath (SOB) but her skin, lips, and nailbeds are pink. Her vital signs are: T: 97.6 (F), P: 110/min., R: 30/min. and deep, BP 148/68, pulse ox: 100%. She admits this has happened before but "never this bad". She says, "I'm not crazy, I know something is wrong with my heart." The physician feels the diagnosis is obvious but orders a chest x-ray, EKG, and ABG's for proof. The chest x-ray is, normal. The EKG is normal except for the fast heart rate. The blood gases are next.

ABG REPORT

Patient: Annie Hood

TEST	RESULT	NORMAL
Hemoglobin:	10 grams	13 female
Hematocrit:	30%	39 female
02 Saturation:	100%	95-100%
p02:	112mmHg	80-100
PH:	7.56	7.35-7.45
pC02	20mmHg	35-45
HC03	20	20-30
COHb	0%	0-1%

Q: Does this patient need blood?

A: No. Remember, females usually have a lower H & H than males. Even though Annie's H & H of 10 grams and 30% is slightly anemic (normal 12 grams and 36%), she's a menstruating female and a vegetarian. That means that she's losing iron every month with her period, and she's not making up for it in her diet. It's easier to get adequate iron from a meat diet than from a vegetable diet. Without iron, you simply can't make hemoglobin molecules to carry oxygen. Annie may need a multivitamin with iron but she doesn't need a transfusion.

Q: Does she need oxygen?

A: No. Her O_2 saturation is a PERFECT 100%. You can't saturate (oxygenate) more than ALL 100% of your hemoglobin. Her pO_2 is high at 112; her skin, lips, and nails are all pink. She does not need oxygen. (see TRIVIA)

TRIVIA: A $5,000,000 NFL wide receiver races 96 yards for a touchdown. He's slightly out of breath, but has a perfect body, a super heart, and a 100% pulse ox. He asks for, and is given, 100% oxygen to breathe for several minutes.

Q: If you can't oxygenate more than 100% of your hemoglobin, why give HIM oxygen?

A: Because he makes $5,000,000 and he can have anything he wants (and that's the only reason).

Q: Is her pH normal?

A: No. Her pH is HIGH at 7.56. Remember: pH is a backwards measure of acidity. A high pH means a LOW acid in her blood.

Q: Is this a respiratory problem?

A: You bet it is! Despite normal oxygen, skin color, EKG, and chest x-ray, she's breathing deep and fast at 30/min. In short, she's OVER-BREATHING (hyperventilating). When she breathes too much, she takes in too much oxygen. Her pO_2 and pulse ox rise. That's a waste of oxygen, but no real problem. But, every overbreath IN ends in an overbreath OUT. That will blow off CO_2 faster than her body can make it. This lowers her pCO_2. Hyperventilating is like shaking a Coca Cola and opening the cap - lots of CO_2 comes out.

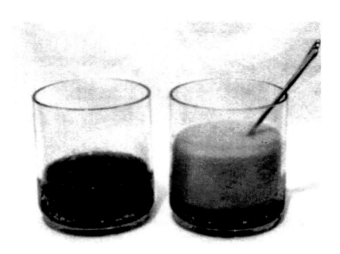

If dissolved CO_2 is acid, then LESS CO_2 is LESS acid. (Higher pH)

Q: Is there a metabolic problem?

A: No. Her HCO_3 (base) is normal at 20. If she continues to over-breathe (hyperventilate) for hours, her kidneys will begin to compensate. They would excrete some more base (HCO_3) to lower her pH. It's too soon for that in the E.R.

Q: What's the ABG diagnosis?

A: This is RESPIRATORY ALKALOSIS. Here's how we got a pH of 7.56. Remember: -

1)Normal pCO_2 (40nm) equals normal pH (7.40).

2)10mm change pCO_2 equals .08 change pH.

3)pCO_2 and pH change in OPPOSITE directions.

So, if a 10mm lower pCO_2 makes the pH rise .08, then Annie's 20mm lower pCO_2 raises the pH by 2 X .08 = 16. So, her ABG's show a pCO_2 of 20 and a pH of 7.56 (7.40 +.16).

Q: What's the diagnosis?

A: Annie has classic hyperventilation syndrome, pure RESPIRATORY ALKALOSIS.

Q: What are we going to do for her?

A: First, be kind. These patients are very frightened. Give her 5-10mg of Valium to calm her. Second, quietly assure her that REBREATHING into a paper bag will help. Why? Each exhale puts CO_2 into the bag. Each inhale then rebreathes the CO_2 until it gradually rises back to normal.

CO_2 concentration has many effects. Too little CO_2 constricts brain arteries causing lightheadedness or fainting. Low CO_2 also lowers calcium in the blood stream. This causes a "short circuit" in nerve impulses and the patient feels numb and tingly. As the CO_2 and calcium continue to fall, painful spasms of the hands and feet make matters worse.

Eventually, the brain stem says, *WHOA!*, and the patient passes out. Breathing stops for 15-20 seconds, CO_2 builds back up in the blood stream, pH falls back to normal, and the patient wakes up. Short term, Annie needs a tranquilizer, a paper bag, and a caring physician or nurse. Long term, she needs stress counseling and possibly medication.

Diabetic Ketoacidosis

Hartley "Hard" Grieves is a 28 year old construction worker. He's a hard living, hard loving, hard drinking, hard smoking, hard working kind of a guy. He's also an insulin-dependent diabetic. Because his disease doesn't fit his image, good diabetic control is not his highest priority.

Hard and his friends just returned from a four-day holiday weekend at the beach. Body abuse seems to have been their main leisure activity. Increased alcohol, decreased sleep, junk food, and irregular insulin doses bring him to the ER today. He's been coughing for two days, vomiting for several hours, and urinating "every five minutes".

His vital signs are T: 100.1 F, P: 120/min., R: 30/min. and deep, BP: 158/96. Pulse ox is 98% but his breath smells like nail polish remover (acetone). He's had these flareups of his diabetes off and on for years. He agrees to " a little tune-up, doc, but lets not take all day".

On physical exam, he has wheezes in his chest and his upper abdomen is tender. His skin is "doughy" when you pinch it. His tongue and lips are dry.

The doctor orders blood tests, ABG's, chest x-ray, urinalysis and an IV wide open. His x-ray is negative. His hemoglobin is 16 and his hematocrit is 48%. Urinalysis shows high sugar and high acetone. Hard lives up to his name with a blood sugar of 758 (more than 7 times normal) and acetone in his blood. His very abnormal blood gases are:

Patient: Hartley Greaves

TEST	RESULT	NORMAL
Hemoglobin:	16 grams	15 male
Hematocrit:	48%	45 male
02 Saturation:	92%	95-100%
p02:	85mmHg	80-100
PH:	7.00	7.35-7.45
pC02	15.5mmHg	35-45
HC03	3.7	20-30
COHb	4%	0-1%

Q: Does Hard need blood?

A: NO. His H & H of 16 grams and 48% is HIGHER than the normal blood count of 14 grams and 40%. So, he doesn't need more blood. The real question is: WHY is his blood count so high?

Q: Okay, why is it high?

A: Because he's dehydrated from out of control diabetes.

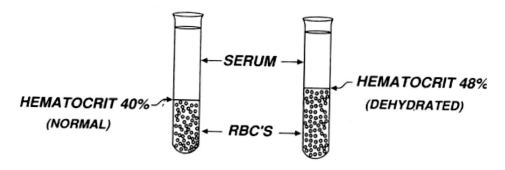

The blood sample on the left has a normal 40% hematocrit. The sample on the right is dehydrated. It has lost some of the LIQUID part of the blood. So the red blood cells make up a bigger part of the sample - a hematocrit of 48%.

Q: Does this patient need oxygen?

A: Yes. The pulse ox of 98% is not correct. The ABG shows the actual O$_2$

saturation is LOW at 92%. He has 4% of his hemoglobin tied up with carbon monoxide (COHb) from his smoking. That's part of the problem with the pulse ox. Also, remember that pulse ox can be off by several percent in either direction.

Q: Is there a respiratory problem?

A: Yes. Somehow he lost most of his pCO_2 ! But his *main* problem is metabolism.

Q: Does he have a METABOLIC problem?

A: Definitely. His bicarb (HCO_3) has dropped all the way from normal (20 to 30) to 3.7! Whoever stole the pCO_2 must have stolen the bicarb as well.

Q: What happened to the bicarbonate?

A: His diabetic keto-ACIDOSIS used it up.

TRIVIA: The reason uncontrolled diabetics become dehydrated is simple. The body likes all its fluids at the same concentration. It wants the same number of chemical particles in each quart of water. Diabetics have a high blood sugar. That means their blood fluid has too many particles in it. (It's too concentrated). This concentrated fluid "sucks" water out of the body's surrounding cells to dilute this sugar - osmosis. That causes two problems. First, the cells begin to dry out from losing their water to the blood stream. Second, the kidneys sense this "extra" water and extra sugar in the blood and increase the urine output.

Q: OK, how did his diabetic ketoacidosis use up his bicarbonate?

NORMAL METABOLISM

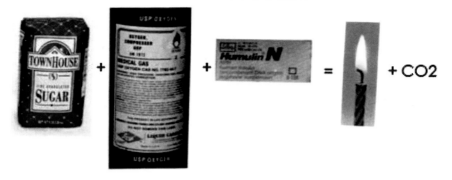

Carbohydrates + Oxygen + Insulin = Energy + CO2

DIABETIC METABOLISM

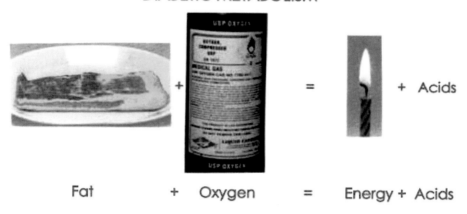

Fat   +   Oxygen   =   Energy + Acids

A: The body needs insulin to burn sugar. Diabetics have little or no insulin. Instead, they burn FAT, sort of like an "alternative fuel". But, alternative fuels often have hidden problems. A body burning fat also produces two ACIDS - acetoacetic acid and hydroxybutyric acid. The patient's bicarb is used to neutralize these extra acids. Respiration then exhales the CO_2 to complete the process.

ACID + BICARB = WATER + CARBON DIOXIDE + ACETONE

$$H^+ + HCO_3^- = H_2O + CO_2 + (acetone)$$

Q: Can we get back to the RESPIRATORY problem?

A: Actually there are two respiratory problems. First, he's breathing fast because he's slightly hypoxic. Why? Because he has fever, cough, and wheezing from his smoker's bronchitis. That won't show up on x-ray. His respirations are also fast trying to exhale the extra CO_2. Remember, the bicarbonate neutralizes acid by converting it to CO_2. That CO_2 MUST be exhaled or it won't compensate.

Q: Why does he smell like nail polish remover?

A: Nail polish remover is acetone. Without insulin he can't burn sugar. So, he burns fat instead. But, burning fat produces the acetone "exhaust" that you smell on his breath.

Q: What's his ABG diagnosis and is he compensating?

A: He has METABOLIC ACIDOSIS. He's trying to compensate with RESPIRATORY ALKALOSIS. With a pH of 7.06 compensation simply isn't working.

Q: What's his medical diagnosis?

A: Acute diabetic ketoacidosis and bronchitis.

Q: What treatment does he need?

A: Bronchitis: First, this needs aerosols for wheezing. Then it needs Tylenol for fever. Finally, it may need antibiotics for infection (most "bronchitis" is viral and viruses don't respond to antibiotics). Extra oxygen will make him more comfortable.

Diabetic ketoacidosis: This is more complicated. He needs insulin to start burning sugar instead of fat. The dehydration needs LOTS of IV fluids - probably 4-5 quarts. Kidney function can usually fix the bicarbonate. But, this very low pH (7.06) and VERY, VERY, LOW bicarbonate 3.7 need help. While it is controversial treatment, extra bicarbonate in his IV may help neutralize more acid by converting it to CO_2- Hard's rapid breathing can then exhale the CO_2 and complete the process.

Legionnaire Pneumonia

Aaron Straight, Jr. is a 38 year old bank vice president known as "Straight Arrow" behind his back. He married his high school sweetheart, has two perfect children (one boy and one girl, of course), and has never smoked or drank. He hasn't had a "sick day" in 17 years at the bank. In the ER today he looks more like he's taking a *dead* day than a *sick* day this time.

For several days he's had the "flu" with cough, muscle aches, and diarrhea. This morning he was so weak from coughing and sweating, he let his wife bring him to the ER. In the lobby he became belligerent and confused.

On the stretcher he is pale, coughing, soaked with sweat, and acutely SOB. His lips and nailbeds are bluish. He's so agitated and confused that he needs to be restrained to be examined. His vital signs are: T: 105.8 F (rectally, since he won't cooperate for an oral temperature), P: 120/min., R: 28/min. and labored from frequent coughing, BP: 102/58, pulse ox: 78% on room air. His left lung sounds congested and almost no breath sounds are heard in his right lung. An EKG shows a fast heart rate and signs of low oxygen to the heart muscle. His chest x-ray shows pneumonia in the left lung and pneumonia and fluid in the right lung. His initial arterial blood gasses are:

ABG REPORT

Patient: Aaron Straight, Jr.

TEST	RESULT	NORMAL
Hemoglobin:	14 grams	15 male
Hematocrit:	42%	45 male
02 Saturation:	77%	95-100%
p02:	50mmHg	80-100
PH:	7.18	7.35-7.45
pC02	60mmHg	35-45
HC03	8	20-30
COHb	0%	0-1%

Q and A

Q: Does this patient need blood?

A: No, with a normal H & H of 14 grams and 42%, that's one of the few normal tests he has.

Q: Does he need oxygen?

A: Immediately! His pO_2 is only 50mm Hg. The oxygen hemoglobin curve shows his O_2 saturation should be about 75%.

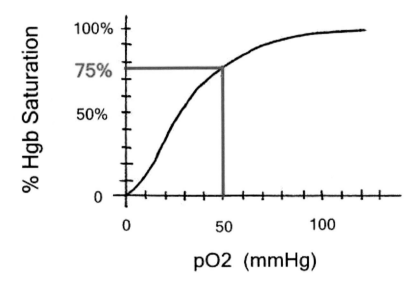

That's pretty close to his ABG O_2 saturation result of 77%. In fact, even his pulse ox "guesstimate" showed only 76% of hemoglobin saturated with oxygen. He needs oxygen - 25% of the blood he's pumping around isn't carrying any. How much oxygen does he need? Don't be stingy. It's plentiful and cheap! Start him at 100% oxygen by using a nonrebreather mask delivering 15 liters/min (see Ways To Add Oxygen).

Q: Does he have a normal pH?

A: At 7.20, his pH is so ACID it's more like lemonade than blood.

Q: Okay, so he's acidotic. Does he have a respiratory problem?

A: For respiratory problems, look at the pCO_2. Aaron's pCO_2 is way UP at 60mm. The question is why. He's breathing hard and fast at 28/min. That should blow off his CO_2. The problem is his pneumonia. The pus in his lungs' air sacs prevents inhaled O_2 from entering the blood. It also prevents blood CO_2 from being exhaled.

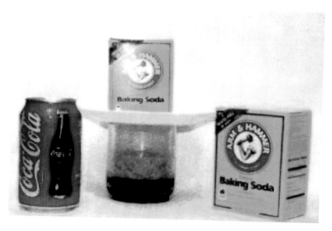

Sort of like shaking a coke bottle with the cap on - there's lots of fizz (CO_2) but it just can't get out.

Q: How about his metabolism - is that a problem as well?

A: His bicarbonate (HCO_3) is way down to 8 (normal 20-30). Yet even with all that bicarbonate neutralizing, he's still acid. Let's calculate why. His pCO_2 is 60mm. That's 20mm above normal. Each 10mm increase in CO_2 LOWERS the pH by .08. So, a 20mm increase in his pCO_2 should only LOWER his pH to 7.24 (7.40 minus (2 x .08) = 7.24). But his pH is 7.18, even LOWER and more ACIDIC than the pCO_2 can account for.

Q: Where's the extra acid coming from?

A: REFRESHER: Normal AEROBIC metabolism means burning sugar with oxygen to make energy. But Aaron doesn't have enough oxygen to burn fuel the usual way. Instead, he's using some *an*aerobic ("no air") metabolism. Remember when the diabetic patient used a different metabolism because he didn't have insulin? That resulted in increased acids (acetoacetic and hydroxybutyric). It also resulted in abnormal "exhaust". Aaron Straight's abnormal ANAEROBIC metabolism is giving him an abnormal exhuast too - LACTIC ACID. That's the source of his additional acidosis. No wonder his poor bicarbonate (HCO_3) is almost gone. Every available HCO_3 is either neutralizing the CO_2 (acid) he's not able to exhale or neutralizing the lactic (acid) his anaerobic metabolism is producing. Is there compensation? : Yes, he's compensating by breathing fast and compensating by trying to hold bicarb, but he's failing.

Q: What's his ABG diagnosis?

A: Severe mixed RESPIRATORY and METABOLIC ACIDOSIS.

Q: What does he need?

A: Poor Mr. Straight has pneumonia in both lungs from Legionnaire's disease. It's so bad he's in respiratory failure. He needs 100% O_2, I.V. antibiotics, and a tube in his windpipe. That will be hooked to a respirator. He simply can't breathe well enough on his own to survive.

NORMAL LUNG 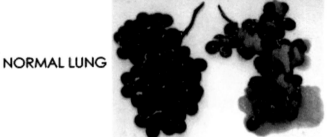 PNEUMONIA LUNG

(Pus & Destruction)

APPENDICES

ABG Tips

1. ABG's are expensive. Depending on the hospital and the part of the country, charges can vary from $50 to over $200 per ABG. Don't order them lightly.

2. ABG's are painful. Otherwise reasonable adults may refuse the test if they've had it before. You make more friends if you first numb the skin with a 27g needle injection of 1% plain lidocaine.

3. ABG's don't need ice. Early data seemed to indicate that ABG results deteriorated with time unless the sample was iced. In fact, if the sample is analyzed in less than 15 minutes, no significant differences occur with or without ice.

4. ABG's can sometimes wait. If you know clinically why the patient is sick (pneumonia, heart failure, asthma, etc.) why not treat the patient first, THEN get the ABG's? Even the patient knew he was sick initially, did you really need ABG's to prove it?

5. ABG's can't rule out a pulmonary embolism (lung blood clot). No single ABG value or combination of values proves a patient does not have an embolism.

6. Pulse ox readings change rapidly. There's no need to wait 20-30 minutes when increasing or decreasing a patient's oxygen. The pulse ox will get better -or worse- in 5 minutes or less.

7. ABG's may not change as rapidly as pulse ox. The pO_2 and O_2 saturation WILL change in less than 5 minutes. But, the acid base changes take longer. Don't expect final changes - or repeat the blood gas - in less than 15-30 minutes.

8. ABG's aren't necessary for carbon monoxide testing. If all you need is the patient's carbon monoxide level, draw the blood from a vein (less painful) not an artery. The other ABG values will be wrong but the COHb will be correct.

Clinical Causes of Acid-Base Problems *

1. METABOLIC ACIDOSIS: COMMON, ↓ pH & ↓ HCO_3
Diabetes
Kidney failure
Lactic acidosis (like exercise)
Poisoning (like aspirin, wood alcohol, and antifreeze)

2. RESPIRATORY ACIDOSIS: COMMON, ↓ pH & ↑ pCO_2
Not breathing (respiratory arrest, narcotic overdose, loss of brain respiratory center)
Blocked breathing (foreign body or tumor in airway)
Can't breathe (crushed chest, paralysis of chest)
Lung failure (pneumonia, asthma, emphysema, lung injury or tumor)

3. RESPIRATORY ALKALOSIS: PRETTY COMMON, ↑ pH & ↓ CO_2
Hyperventilation syndrome
Fever
Hypoxia
Improper setting on mechanical ventilator
Brain problem (overstimulating respiratory center)
Liver failure

4. METABOLIC ALKALOSIS: UNCOMMON, ↑ pH & ↑ HCO_3
Vomiting (loss of stomach acid)
Diuretics (complex mechanism)
Too much cortisone (from body or medication - very complex mechanism)

* Common causes - by NO means a complete list!

Age Corrected pO_2

Two bits of news about aging are helpful. First the bad news: your **normal** pO_2 gets lower each year you're alive. But, the good news is it's probably the ONLY part of the aging process you won't notice!

How low can the pO_2 be and still be normal for your age? Since nobody really knows, they've created lots of complex formulas factoring in age, height above sea level, patient position (lying? sitting? standing?), etc.

Actually, the best "guesstimate" is below. The normal pO_2 drops about 5 mm for each 10 years:

$$30 \text{ years} = 95 \text{ mm } pO_2$$
$$40 \text{ years} = 90 \text{ mm } pO_2$$
$$50 \text{ years} = 85 \text{ mm } pO_2$$
$$60 \text{ years} = 80 \text{ mm } pO_2$$
$$70 \text{ years} = 75 \text{ mm } pO_2$$
$$80 \text{ years} = 70 \text{ mm } pO_2$$

After 80 years, if you're not short of breath, and you're still alive, you're doing just fine!

Q: How can a pO_2 of only 70mm be OK?

A: Remember that the Oxy/Hgb Dissociation Curve is a curve and not a straight line. Remember the orange highlighted "safety" area of the Oxy/Hgb Curve? That allows good oxygen saturation even at a slightly lower pO_2 as we age.

Ways to Add Oxygen

The air we breathe is about 21% oxygen. If the patient needs more oxygen here are 5 choices:

METHOD	OXYGEN	APPROXIMATE % OF OXYGEN PATIENT GETS
1. Nasal Prongs	2-4 liters/min	25-30 %
2. Face Mask	5-6 liters/min	40 %
3. Non-rebreathing mask	15 liters/min	95 %
4. Veni mask	varies	25-50 %
5. Mechanical Ventilator	50 P.S.I.	21-100 %

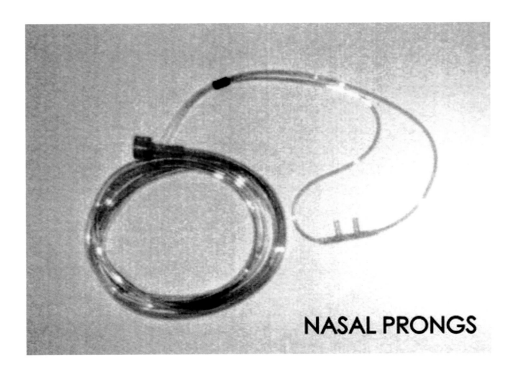

NASAL PRONGS

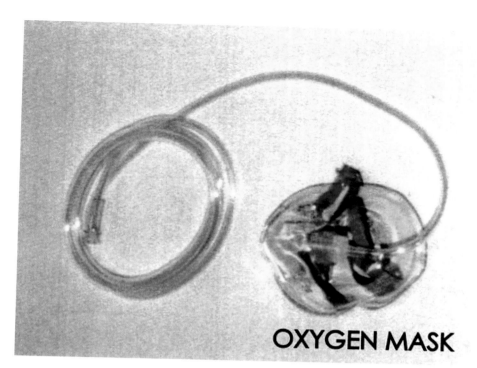

OXYGEN MASK

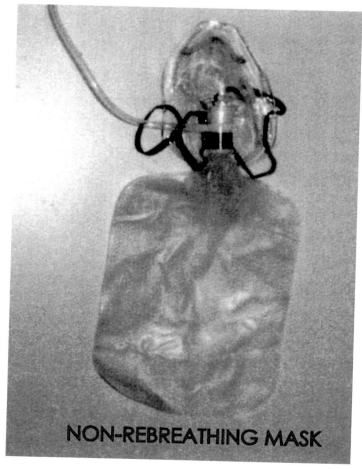

NON-REBREATHING MASK

VENTURI MASK

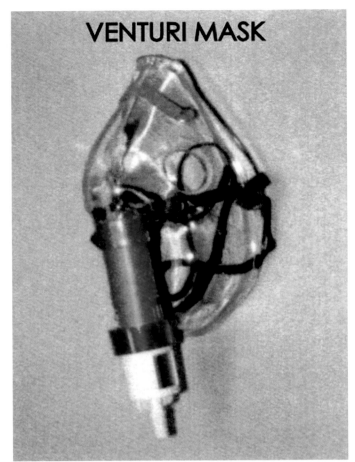

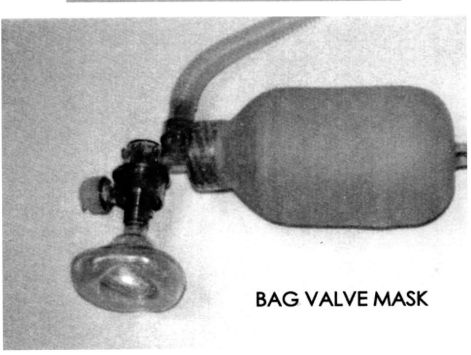

BAG VALVE MASK

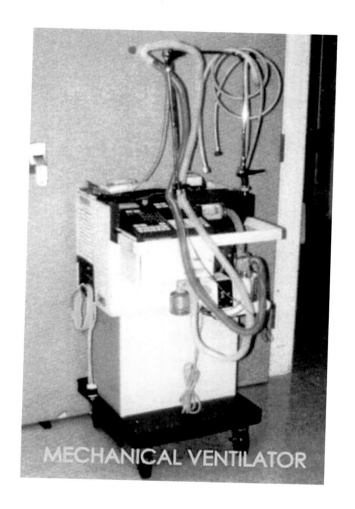

MECHANICAL VENTILATOR

Shifting The Curve

UNFORTUNATELY, the oxyhemoglobin dissociation curve is not written in stone. The curve can slide to the right or to the left on the graph. FORTUNATELY, these effects are mostly seen in extreme cases (and beyond the scope of a primer like <u>Simple as ABG</u>). Correction of the underlying problem usually shifts the curve back in place.

1. SHIFTS TO THE RIGHT

The shift can be caused by: fever, anemia, hypoxia, acidosis.

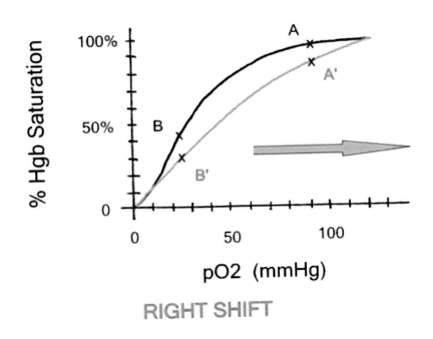

RIGHT SHIFT

This shift means Hgb picks up LESS oxygen in the lungs (A vs A') but releases oxygen MORE easily at the tissues' (B vs B'). This is helpful in very sick patients.

2. SHIFTS TO THE LEFT

The shift can be caused by: hypothermia, alkalosis.

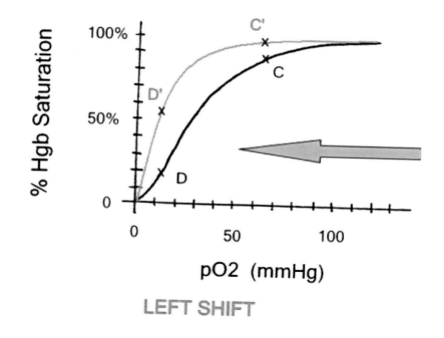

LEFT SHIFT

Left shift does the opposite of right. At high pO2's (like 80mm), MORE Hgb will be bound to oxygen (C vs C'). At low pO2's (like 20mm), LESS oxygen will be released from Hgb to the tissues (D vs D'). This is not helpful in very sick patients, but is also rare.

The A-a Gradient

Academic physicians insist that ABG's are too complicated to be simplified. This belief is very apparent in the A-a gradient. What's that you ask? It's the difference between the amount of oxygen in the artery (A) and the amount of oxygen in the alveoli (a) . This "simple" calculation is supposedly useful in clinical practice. Here are three reasons why I've left it out.

(1) It's NOT a simple calculation. The actual formula is:

$$FiO_2 \times (Pbar - pH2O) - (pCO_2/R) - pO_2 = \text{A-a Gradient}$$

It's "simplified" to be:

$$150 - (pO_2 + pCO_2) = \text{A-a Gradient}$$

Now, the normal pO_2, normal pCO_2, and even the "normal" A-a gradient vary with patient age, supplemental O_2 , height above sea level, whether the patient is lying down or sitting up, past and present disease, etc. The short formula conveniently ignores these variations completely.

(2) It's NOT a good screening test for blood clots in the lung (pulmonary embolism) . It seems if oxygen gets into the lungs (a) but not into the artery (A), the artery must be blocked. Right? WRONG. The P.I.O.P.E.D. study (Prospective Investigation of Pulmonary Embolism Diagnosis) is one of many studies proving the A-a gradient is very unreliable. Missing 20% of patients with blood clots seems like a bad idea to me.

(3) In 35 years of ER experience I have never seen a physician make a diagnostic or therapeutic decision based on the A-a gradient. Ask your doctor the last time he or she did the math. Don't be surprised if you get a blank stare!

Simple as ABG

———◆———